GIFT OF ANOTHER
Breath
YOU HAVE PANCREATIC CANCER

Angella Dixon-Watson

ISBN 978-1-64003-458-7 (Paperback)
ISBN 978-1-64003-459-4 (Digital)

Copyright © 2017 Angella Dixon-Watson
All rights reserved
First Edition

All rights reserved. No part of this publication may be reproduced, distributed, or transmitted in any form or by any means, including photocopying, recording, or other electronic or mechanical methods without the prior written permission of the publisher. For permission requests, solicit the publisher via the address below.

Covenant Books, Inc.
11661 Hwy 707
Murrells Inlet, SC 29576
www.covenantbooks.com

Contents

My Journey 7
Endoscopy 9
Reality Check 10
Warfare Arsenal 12
Whipple Surgery to Remove Duodenal Adenocarcinoma ... 14
Home Recovery 16
The Diagnosis 21
Fellowship with Friends 22
Coping with the Diagnosis 31
Anticipating Chemo Regiment 33
Chemo Regiment 35
Cancer Free 42
Encouragements in Different Ways 45
Moving Forward 49
Diet 51
Continuing Activities 52
Remembrance 53
Healing Scriptures 55

Additional Comforting Scriptures 56

Acknowledgments 59

Encouragements 63

Nurturing Praise and Worship Songs that Ministered to my Soul.....65

Cast All Your Care on Him

Cast all your care on Him
Cast all your care on Him
For He cares for you
He died for you
Cast all your care on Him

Cast all your hope on Him
Cast all your hope on Him
For He feels your pain
He knows your name
Cast all your hope on Him

Jesus sees every sparrow
He will quench the fiery arrows
Jesus didn't bring you this far
Just to leave you now

Cast all your fear on Him
Cast all your hope on him
For He cares for you
Spilled blood for you
Cast all your care on Him

(Words and Music by Ira Watson)

MY JOURNEY

Charity Function

It was a beautiful Saturday evening on April 23, 2016, when I attended a fundraising event in Wheaton, Maryland, in support of the Mustard Seed Communities.

The Mustard Seed organization helps the most vulnerable in Jamaica. There are limited facilities, governmental or otherwise, available to take care of individuals with mental and physical disabilities after the age of eighteen. One of my passions is to support agencies that provide care to children and adults with varying kinds of disabilities (intellectual and developmental). And here is why. My daughter, Raquel-Ann, was born with cerebral palsy. She is now in her 30's and is totally dependent. I am blessed to have the support of Caroline Center's community day program, Burtonsville, and the ARC of Prince Georges County, Maryland, residential managed care. In most developing countries, this support is non-existent. The function was well attended. Island music was jamming, and to top it off, they served Jamaican black fruit cake and great Caribbean food. What a joyful evening!

Benchmark

Well, the following week after the event, I started experiencing itching in the palm of my hands. There is a myth in the islands, when this happens, *money is on the way*. Well, that did not happen. The itching became more severe toward the end of April; and by early May 2016, I realized that I was becoming extremely jaundiced and was rapidly losing weight. This was not normal. So within three weeks, symptoms became more severe, such as I could not sleep at nights. My husband, Ira, said he heard me crying out in bed due to the pain from the itching and scratching. One day, he had a concerned look on his face and said to me, "Are you losing weight?"

When I had my annual checkup in March 2016 with my primary-care physician, my weight was 164 pounds. And it was now visible that something strange was happening to me physically.

Fortunately, the extreme itching graduated to my arms and then my entire body, except my face. Why do I say fortunately? If it were not for the severe itching, scratching, rapid weight loss, sleepless nights, and extreme jaundiced situation, I may have taken the matter lightly, thinking it might be allergies; but since I don't suffer from allergies, I knew I'd better get checked out.

Due to the symptoms, I visited my primary-care physician in May. Lab tests were performed and vitals were taken; and the report came back as abnormal liver tests. In March, when I saw that same doctor as part of my annual physical checkup, I was in perfect health. So what was really happening here?

After my primary-care physician saw the results of the lab work, she immediately referred me to Capital Digestive Care and I made an appointment. More labs and scans were done. The scans results came back showing that there was a cyst, but the kind of cyst that was unknown (cancerous or noncancerous). Before the type of cyst was identified as cancerous, my childhood friend Esther shared my health challenges with her unofficially adopted daughter, Betty Jean, a fasting and praying person.

BJ sensed danger and called me from Texas with urgency in her voice. Her words were, "Take communion three times daily. Use whatever juice you have at home. Also, don't eat anything white, such as pasta and rice."

Wow! These words were a shocker. And I tried my best to adhere to those words—although not perfectly.

The diagnosis said, "Acute hepatitis and choledochal cyst." So an endoscopy was ordered.

ENDOSCOPY

I had the endoscopy on May 31, 2016, at the University of Maryland, Baltimore. After the endoscopy, we were told that I had duodenal adenocarcinoma.

What is duodenal adenocarcinoma?

Duodenal adenocarcinoma is a cancer in the beginning section of the small intestine. It is relatively rare compared to gastric cancer and colorectal cancer.

When I was in the recovery room after the endoscopy, the surgeon told me that they placed a stent in the bile duct. Then I said, "So I will come back in two weeks and you'll get it out."

The doctor looked puzzled.

Concerned about the yellowing of my eyes, I asked, "Will I get my eyes back?"

He said, "Yes, the jaundiced situation will clear up." All this time he kept looking at Ira and said, "You didn't tell her." The doctor had already consulted with him.

Ira replied, "I want her to hear it from you."

The physician then said, "You have cancer. However, because of the location, it *is* curable. The cancer had not penetrated any organs." Hearing the word *curable* relieved some of my stress and anxiety, and we were hopeful. Whipple surgery for duodenal adenocarcinoma was scheduled for Thursday, June 30.

REALITY CHECK

I got my paperwork in order. I also typed a draft of "Celebrating the life of" program outlining format, songs, minister, and who should be in charge of coordinating my possible "good bye" service. I did these things so that Ira would not be extremely stressed if duodenal adenocarcinoma surgery was unsuccessful.

Okay, what have I learned up to this point:

First, listen to your body. It speaks to you.

Second, don't hesitate going to see your primary-care physician if in doubt about unusual symptoms. I did not need to get a second opinion, but feel free to do so if your spirit tells you.

Third, I got my advance directives in order, which would make it less stressful on the family.

Fourth, my life changed within four weeks. If I had ignored the severe itching, extreme jaundice, and rapid weight loss, I would have missed the opportunity to share my story detailing God's grace and mercy. My hope is that my story will encourage others who may get a terminally ill diagnosis and may be unsure of the final outcome.

> I will lift up mine eyes unto the hills, from whence cometh my help.
> My help cometh from the Lord, which made heaven and earth.
> He will not suffer thy foot to be moved; he that keeps you will not slumber.
> Behold, he that keeps Israel shall neither slumber nor sleep.
> The Lord is thy keeper: the Lord is thy shade upon thy right hand.

GIFT OF ANOTHER BREATH

The sun shall not smite you by day, nor the moon by night.
The Lord shall preserve you from all evil: he shall preserve thy soul.
The Lord shall preserve thy going out and thy coming in from this time forth,
and even for evermore. (Ps.121)

WARFARE ARSENAL

For God hath not given us a spirit of fear
But of power, and of love and of a sound mind. (2 Tim.1:7)

In light of the information I received, I realized that I could not go this journey alone. As a result, I engaged in primarily two activities: I watched "faith and believe" based non-denominational preachers on television and was reminded of the importance of *"speaking positive words over my life" and this became my daily formula. In addition, I ordered the following items online:*

- CDs loaded with healing songs from SonLife Broadcasting Network (SBN)
- CD with healing scriptures spoken by Kenneth Copeland
- Dodi Osteen's book *Healed of Cancer*

The Story of a Liver Cancer Survivor

I felt a connection to Dodi Osteen's story, and here is why: She was unable to sleep, became weak and jaundiced, lost weight quickly—similar symptoms I experienced. And believe it or not, she had a daughter who was born with cerebral palsy, just like my daughter, Raquel-Ann.

While reading her story, I learned not to come in agreement with fear. Neither give place to the devil. (Eph. 4:27)

I learned to fight my battles with the enemy by using the word of God. I walked around my home openly repeating the following:

GIFT OF ANOTHER BREATH

Enemy, you wanted to take me out
silently but God Stopped you
He made me experienced severe itching
which I had to scratch so hard
I felt as if I wanted to take off my skin.
You failed because God has plans for my life!

Put on the whole armour of God, that ye may be able to stand against the wiles of the devil. For we wrestle not against flesh and blood, but against principalities, against powers, against the rulers of the darkness of this world, against spiritual wickedness in high places. (Eph. 6:11–12)

WHIPPLE SURGERY TO REMOVE DUODENAL ADENOCARCINOMA

What is Whipple surgery?

This surgery removes part of the pancreas, the small intestine, stomach, bile duct, and all of the gall bladder. As a result of this kind of surgery, the amount of food one can consume changes, along with the way food is metabolized.

Upcoming surgery
June 30, 2016

Friends offered to be at the hospital with me in support of Ira. Some said that they wanted to represent my mom, Bobsie I. Evans-Shirley, affectionately called Ms. Babs, who passed unexpectedly on December 29, 2009. She was a cosmetologist; business owner; and much loved. She had a heart full of kindness and love for all, which was a gift she received from her mother, Lurline Dwyer-Marlin. Both are greatly missed by family and friends.

Whipple surgery was performed on Thursday, June 30, and lasted up to five hours. The hospital preferred that not more than two people at a time should visit me in the recovery room after surgery. Two of my old friends and former work colleagues, Paulette and Jennifer, World Bank retirees, came on the day of the surgery along with Ira. My son Dino and my daughter-in-law Cristy also joined the group. The waiting area was known as the Healing Garden; it had a large open glass enclosure to the sky, with palm trees and exotic plants everywhere. Healing Garden—how appropriately named. So after surgery, my visitors took turns (two by two) seeing me in the recovery room.

The surgery went well, and specimens were sent to the lab. The lab report came back stating that cancer had penetrated the pancreas and was in four of the thirteen lymph nodes. All this was unknown to me while staying in the hospital for almost two weeks, and also during recovery at home. I am grateful that I did not know the lab results during this time—not sure I would have had the will to be strong.

So if I did not have surgery for duodenal adenocarcinoma, pancreatic cancer would possibly be discovered at a later date, and that would definitely not be good.

> As for you, you meant evil against me, but God meant it for good, to bring it about that many people should be kept alive, as they are today. (Gen. 50:20)

> Fear thou not, for I am with thee; be not dismayed; for I am thy God I will strengthen thee; yea. I will help thee, yea I will uphold thee with the right hand of my righteousness. (Isa. 41:10)

The University of Maryland Hospital, Baltimore, has a great staff. And while on the fifth floor for twelve days, I became attached to Nurse Tierra, whose mannerisms and kindness reminded me of my friend Carolyn, who is a nurse down South. What should have been a week's stay, however, ended up being almost two weeks. I received bouquets, many visitors, and countless telephone calls and texts, for which I am extremely grateful. I was discharged Tuesday, July 12.

HOME RECOVERY

> Beloved, I wish above all things that you prosper and
> be in health, even as thy soul prospers. (John 3:2)

Thanks be to God, the duodenal adenocarcinoma surgery was successful. I was home recovering and remained positive. So I was looking forward to my follow-up visit in two weeks to be told that I was *cancer free*.

"You have pancreatic cancer"

My follow-up visit was two weeks later, on July 27, and that morning I was excited. I believed that I would get a clean bill of health. So Ira and I headed off to the hospital, and we met with the surgeon who performed the Whipple surgery for duodenal adenocarcinoma. The surgeon entered the room and sat on a chair to the left of me, with the lab report in his hands. He said *slowly* and *compassionately*, "The cancer has penetrated the pancreas. It's slightly aggressive. Four out of thirteen nodes were checked, and the cancer was found in four of the nodes. The news felt like a hurricane and tornado all in one!"

The surgeon also said that he would set up an appointment for me to meet with the oncology team.

I remember saying to him, "Let me put on my glasses so I can read the report." Of course, I did not understand much of what I was reading. I continued reading the lab report, and I came across words like *neuroendocrine tumor, perineural invasion, and pathologic tumor stage: pt 3 ni mx*. I then said to myself, *I wonder if this means stage 3.*

The surgeon had already left the room, and I said to Ira, we forgot to ask the stage. So we asked a nurse who was passing by the consultation room to find out from the surgeon what stage it was. The answer came back: *stage 2*.

Unfortunately, news of getting a clean bill of health was not the case during my follow-up appointment. Imagine that, within a four-week period—between May 31, 2016, and June 30, 2016—the cancer had penetrated the pancreas and the lymph nodes in such a short space of time.

A member of the medical team encouraged me not to do Google searches on pancreatic cancer since the data I find may be outdated and discouraging.

> Guard your heart above all else for it determines the course of your life. (Prov. 4:23)

These words reminded me to meditate on things that bring good report. As you know, a ship does not sink based on the water around it. It sinks when the water gets into it.

After the meeting with the surgeon, my mind started racing; and the first thing I said to myself was, How am I going to tell our son, Dino, this news? And I will also have to tell our daughter, Raquel-Ann. Writing this section has made me relive that day in July when my life and Ira's life changed. He instantly became a primary caregiver.

> For I will restore health unto thee, and I will heal thee of thy wounds, saith the Lord… (Jer. 30:17)

> Many are the afflictions of the righteous; But the Lord delivers him out of them all. (Ps. 34:19)

> Heal me, LORD, and I will be healed; save me and I will be saved, for you are the one I praise. (Jer. 17:14)

> Yet I still dare to hope when I remember this. The faithful love of the LORD never ends! His mercies never cease. Great is his faithfulness; his mercies begin

afresh each morning. I say to myself, "The LORD is my inheritance; therefore, I will hope in him!" The LORD is good to those who depend on him, to those who search for him. (Lam. 3:21–25)

What have I learned up to this point?

The family going through a life-changing event does not think clearly during medical consultations. They are still in shock. For example, Ira and I forgot to ask what stage was the cancer.

Meeting the Oncology Team

Tuesday, August 2, 2016

They separately explained the next steps in treatment protocol, which were chemo for six months and then radiation when chemo ended. And it was up to me to decide if I wanted to proceed with treatment. I expressed that I knew no one who survived pancreatic cancer, and I was hesitant to consider taking any treatment. I asked, if I did not do treatment, how many months would I have?

The doctor looked at the chart on the computer and then said six months.

Regarding radiation, I was given the option to be a part of a study. However, if I participated in the study, there was no guarantee that I would be chosen for radiation. And I wanted to keep my options open. In addition, the decision to do radiation was not necessary for me to make at that time since that treatment would start after completing six months of chemotherapy. Incidentally, chemo lasted seven and a half months instead, and here is why: when the scheduled chemo treatment for six months ended, I started radiation and chemo together for an additional five and a half weeks.

After the consultations ended regarding next treatment steps, a scan was ordered that would help to establish the benchmark for chemo treatment. The scan result came back and showed that there was no further spread and I was encouraged. So I signed the agreement to move ahead with treatment.

Because I decided to move forward with chemo, on Tuesday, August 9, a portacath was inserted into my upper left shoulder.

What is a portacath?

A *portacath* is an implanted venous access device for patients who need frequent or continuous administration of chemotherapy. Drugs used for chemotherapy are often toxic and can damage skin, muscle tissue, and sometimes veins.

My veins are not the best, and the portacath would make it less painful for me to do labs and easier to receive chemo infusion every Tuesday in Baltimore.

What have I learned?

First, don't assume that you will experience the side effects that others experienced. Due to the fear of the unknown, I almost walked away from starting treatment and I would have been gone within six months.

Second, going ahead with a holistic approach, chemotherapy, or radiation therapy is an individual decision. And I understand that there are other treatment options available.

Third, you must accept the outcome of your decision regarding type of treatment.

At some point, I started wondering, Why is pancreatic cancer so hard to be detected early? So at the end of my seven-and-a-half-month treatment protocol (increased from six months), I did a Google search on that subject and got the following information from the site of the American Cancer Society.

Can pancreatic cancer be found early?

Pancreatic cancer is hard to find early. The pancreas is deep inside the body, so early tumors can't be seen or felt by health care providers during routine physical exams. People usually have no symptoms until the cancer has already spread to other organs.

Screening tests or exams are used to look for a disease in people who have no symptoms (and who have not had that disease before). At this time, no major professional groups recommend routine screening for pancreatic cancer in people who are at average risk. This is because no screening test has been shown to lower the risk of dying from this cancer.

Sometimes when a person has pancreatic cancer, the levels of certain proteins in the blood go up. These proteins, called *tumor markers*, can be detected with blood tests. The tumor markers CA 19-9 and carcinoembryonic antigen (CEA) are the ones most closely tied to pancreatic cancer. But these proteins don't always go up when a person has pancreatic cancer; and even if they do, the cancer is often already advanced by the time this happens.

Sometimes levels of these tumor markers can go up even when a person doesn't have pancreatic cancer.

For these reasons, blood tests aren't used to screen for pancreatic cancer, although a doctor might still order these tests if a person has symptoms that might be from pancreatic cancer. These tests are more often used in people already diagnosed with pancreatic cancer to help tell if treatment is working or if the cancer is progressing.

THE DIAGNOSIS

Prior to going into the hospital for duodenal adenocarcinoma surgery (not pancreatic cancer surgery), I shared with only a few friends and family of my upcoming surgery scheduled for June 30. I truly believed that I would be cancer free after surgery and there would be no need to tell them my illness.

However, the tide had changed, and with this serious diagnosis of pancreatic cancer, I shared with more family and friends; and the word got around, which resulted in beautiful fellowships at home through visits and intercessory prayers.

FELLOWSHIP WITH FRIENDS

Impromptu anointing

On a home visit, my friends Uva and Frank performed an anointing on me. I did not have olive oil, and so we used organic coconut oil from the kitchen. Prayer was offered, and I felt God's presence.

> Is any sick among you? Let him call for the elders of the church; And let them pray over him, anointing him with oil in the name of the Lord. (James 5:14)

Impromptu Intercessory Prayer

I also have to mention this experience. On Sunday, September 4, my friend Marva had a birthday celebration. And during her welcome talk, she mentioned that I was about to start chemo in a day or two. To my surprise, a friend of hers said, "Let's pray for her right now." And yes, the birthday celebration shifted slightly into a prayer session.

> As you help us by your prayers, then many will give thanks on our behalf for the gracious favor granted us in answer to the prayers of many. (2 Cor. 1:11)

Surprise Out-of-Town Visitors

On a Saturday afternoon in August, local friends came by to fellowship. And one of them, Joy, gifted me a beautiful Royal Albert tea set. She then read the story of the potter and the clay and explained how the set was made in the refinery. The emphasis was that God is the potter and I am the clay. He will mold me into a flawless piece of work for his glory. "Yet you, LORD, are our Father. We are the clay, you are the potter; we are all the work of your hand" (Isa. 64:8).

Shortly after her words of encouragement, there was a knock on my front door and there stood my friend, Esther, with a bouquet covering her face. She left Orlando, Florida; drove about fifteen hours to visit me; and then drove back to Florida the following day. Later that evening, there was a severe thunderstorm; and yes, two more out-of-town visitors came, and they were cousins Pansy and Nicole. It was an evening of songs and intercessory prayers.

Another big surprise visit was the following day, Sunday, when my friend Bertram came by with Pastor Frazier and family, who were visiting the area. Prayer was once again offered for my healing.

Friday-Evening Meditation

Two Friday evenings Donna-Marie and Winston came by, and we fellowshipped over supper, and I had the privilege to speak with her mom (Mother Darlington) in Tobago, who had me prayed up. *The* theme on one of the evenings was on *healing balm*. I shared with them that the healing balm topic was no coincidence since I recently heard a sermon by Pastor Novella Smith referencing "healing balm". The sermon encouraged my soul, brought hope and I cried out quietly to my heavenly father and claimed healing. I heard the sermon shortly after I started my chemo regiment and had many more months to go. The thrust of the fellowship was that God still cares and heals. Thankfully, my faith and believe journey started strengthening about 3 years ago and it helped me to understand the significance of anointing; story of the potter and the clay; visitations; healing balm; meditation and prayers.

Visitations

Visits came in different formats, such as physical home checks, phone calls, and texts. I borrowed encouraging words from two of my text visitors and shared the quotes with others: Nedra's "Prayers ascending" and Iying's daily scriptures, which were always so timely on Tuesdays while I sat in the chemo chair. For example,

Blessings

(Gem for the Day)

October 25, 2016

> Yet in all these things, we are more than conquerors
> Through him who loved us
> For I am persuaded that neither death nor life
> Nor angels nor principalities nor powers nor things present nor
> Things to come nor height nor depth nor any other created thing, shall be
> able to separate us from the love of God which is in Christ Jesus
> (Rom. 8: 37–39)

As you praise God today, write out a list of the Lord's blessings and allow your heart to soar in gratitude as you thank him. Enjoy this beautiful day!

Sometimes, to take my mind off daily chemo regiment, I accompanied my friend Salome to a local eatery, where we treated ourselves to one of their nutritious salads and organic drinks. While relaxing, we engaged in lots of laughter! I also have cherished memories hanging out at eateries on separate occasions with friends Sandy, Christiana, Winsome and daughter Trudy; and cousin Nicole.

I received weekly gorgeous and stunningly beautiful electronic bouquets from my friend Mary, with a note saying "Hugs."

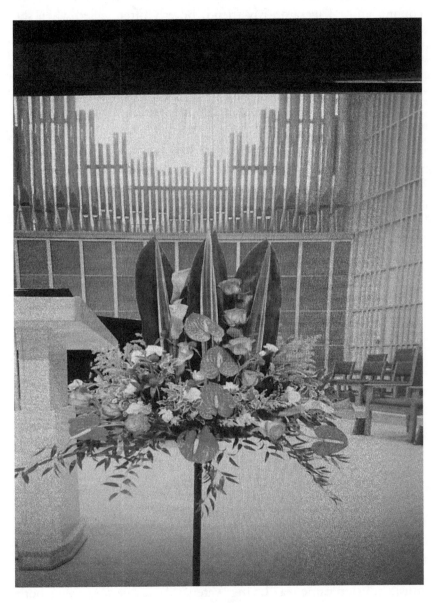

"Hugs"

Friends brought organic and non organic items; such as juices, fruits, flaxseed, chia, vegetables and teas, which flooded my kitchen counter and refrigerator. My friend, Beverly often called when she was heading to the grocery store and her words were: Angie do you need anything? Another friend, Gwen, brought me ready to eat tasty vegetarian meatballs that were gifted to me from friends of hers. While witnessing such kindness from everyone, apart from saying thank you aloud, I whispered under my breath "they want me to live."

When I lived in North Carolina, my two buddies were Carolyn and Charlene. And, since I returned to Maryland we have kept in close contact and they have been a source of consolace during my health journey. In addition, while in NC, I met a beautiful senior lady, Ms. Verona. I call her "beauty". Ever since we met, she always had me prayed up. And, if she called and did not get me, she would sing or left a prayer on my phone. One of her favorite songs was "It is well with my soul."

Ira often asked, "Angie, how do you know so many people?"

I laughed and said, "By being friendly over the years!"

He marveled that friends surprised me with so many visits, new outfits to fit my reduced body frame (pajama set came in the mail) from Judith in Florida and another, Judy from Florida, mailed me soursop leaves, which is used as a herbal tea.

In addition, I was made aware that friends (Cassette and Olive) submitted my name to prayer groups locally and nationally. In early 2017, I became attached to one of the prayer groups out of New Jersey, Church of the Oranges. My friend, Winsome submitted my name, and I tapped into their early morning (6:00 a.m.) prayer line. It so happens that SonLife Broadcasting Network (SBN) aired on TV at the same time. And I was able to listen to intercessory prayers on the prayer line and at the same time got encouraged by the music of the praise and worship team of (SBN). In the evenings at 3pm, my music infusion came via "Living Waters" SBN. The songs were both gospel and hymns—what a treat!

God's Army Supported the Prayer Warriors

The encouragement below is for all prayer warriors. I do not know everyone. I am grateful that you interceded to God on my behalf by *"standing in the gap."* I hope the following words encourage you:

> Speaking to one another in psalms and hymns and spiritual songs, singing and making melody with your heart to the Lord; Always giving thanks to God the Father for everything in the name of our Lord Jesus Christ. (Eph. 5:19)

Here is a biblical success story of the importance of "standing in the gap by praying for others," and it's about Peter who was thrown in prison by Herod, and he was asleep when a miracle happened (Acts 12:1–11). While in prison, friends were praying for him. Suddenly, an angel of the Lord appeared, and a light shone in the cell. He shook Peter and woke him up. "Quick, get up!" he said, and the chains fell off of Peter's wrists.

Do you also recall the story of Elisha when he was surrounded by the Syrian Army. His servant told him that they were going to be destroyed.

> And Elisha prayed, "Open his eyes, LORD, so that he may see." Then the LORD opened the servant's eyes, and he looked and saw the hills full of horses and chariots of fire all around Elisha. (2 Kings 6:17)

I now understand the impact of intercessory prayer. You are not alone, the army of God comes to the rescue.

> Therefore encourage one another and build up one another, just as you also are doing. (1 Thess. 5:11)

> "Do not neglect to do good and to share what you have, for such sacrifices are pleasing to God. (Heb. **13:16**)

ANGELLA DIXON-WATSON

*Let no one seek his own good, but that
of his neighbor. (1 Cor. 10:24)*

Grandkids Cierra and Chase hand-made Get-well notes for me, which I posted on a red background poster and pinned on the wall. Those words encouraged me to continue to believe God for my healing. Cristy, daughter–in-law, was always supportive.

Dino, son, poured out his heart on Facebook, and that was his way of dealing with the news of my health situation. Raquel-Ann, daughter, may have used the same format if it were possible for her to do so.

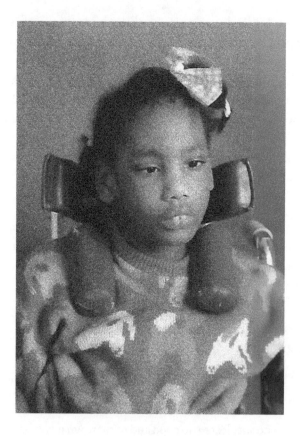

"Raquel-Ann"
Daughter

GIFT OF ANOTHER BREATH

My family in Mexico kept me prayed up as well, and my father, Dorel Dixon, former athlete — Mr. Jamaica; winner of World Wrestling titles and currently a health and fitness advocate — diligently kept in touch with his "first born." He called me from Puebla many times each week. His mother, my grandmother Eunice Walker-Spencer, loved to sing, and he got the gift from her. Oftentimes, he sang to me "Beautiful flowers, beautiful flowers, be like morning dew, beautiful flowers, beautiful flowers you can be like Him."

And, here is another song:

>Blow me a kiss from across the room
>Say I look nice when I'm not
>Touch my hair as you pass my chair
>Little things mean a lot
>Give me your arm as we cross the street
>Call me at six on the dot
>A line a day when you're far away
>Little things mean a lot
>Don't have to buy me diamonds and pearls
>Champagne, sables, or such
>I never cared much for diamonds and pearls
>'Cause honestly, honey, they just cost money
>Give me your hand when I've lost the way
>Give me your shoulder to cry on
>Whether the day is bright or gray
>Give me your heart to rely on
>Send me the warmth of a secret smile
>To show me you haven't forgot
>For always and ever, now and forever
>Little things mean a lot
>Give me your hand when I've lost the way
>Give me your shoulder to cry on
>Whether the day is bright or gray
>Give me your heart to rely on
>Send me the warmth of a secret smile
>To show me you haven't forgot
>That always and ever, now and forever
>Little things mean a lot

My mother's friends were constantly checking in on my progress (Misses Thelma, Nola, Beulah, Jackson, Isaacs, Phil, Cindy, Lascelle [affectionately called Limbo]) and my stepfather, Mr. Deny.

Received calls of encouragements from my mother's unofficially adopted sons, Anah and Edmond; relatives Aunt Phyllis, Uncles Lloyd and Winston, Yvette, Paul, Corey, Westney, Ms. Rose, and Bobby all live outside of the United States.

May these words comfort you.

> May the God of Peace consecrate you through and through! Spirit, soul, and body, may you be kept without break or blame Till the arrival of our Lord Jesus Christ! He who calls you is faithful he will do this. (1 Thess. 5:23–24, Moffat)

During this journey, I often reminisced about my aunt Nesta, and I missed our weekly Sunday morning chit chatting sessions. She would have been another source of encouragement if she were still with us. Also missed are my grandfathers Kenneth George Spencer (a praying person) and Edward Steven Evans (Teddy); fun loving and who often asked: how is the little girl--- referencing great grand daughter, Raquel-Ann.

Another person who had blessed me with great advice for many years and who would have "bathed" me in prayer if she were still with us was mother, Ottley. Apart from our phone conversations when I lived in North Carolina, I also received a letter in my mailbox.

What was enforced up to this point were the following:

First, prayer works, and God's army comes as reinforcement.

Second, it is okay to share your diagnosis with people you trust.

Third, be thankful for all forms of love, such as home visits, homemade meals, visits by e-mail, texts, or phone calls.

Fourth, consider yourself blessed when you are prayed for because some people are less fortunate.

COPING WITH THE DIAGNOSIS

"Know Your Body"

Although the diagnosis was life-threatening, I tried not to panic. I knew that I could not start chemo immediately, which would have started in August instead of September, and here is why. Between May and August, I had already lost 36.6 pounds (164 lbs to 127.4 lbs) and was still recuperating from the Whipple surgery, which lasted for up to five hours. While at home, I had to gradually introduce my body to food and try to eat as consistently as possible. There was no way I would have survived daily treatments of oral chemo and weekly treatment of chemo infusion for the next six months. And, in the end, it turned out that I did chemo for seven and a half months instead of six months.

Before I agreed to move ahead with chemotherapy, someone from the nursing team went over the paperwork and rattled off the side effects of chemotherapy. Hearing the side effects placed me in a melancholy state, wondering if I should be bothered with treatment.

Although my situation was grave, I asked the oncologist to give me time to build up my body through nutrition. Thankfully, I was given about three weeks to do so. As a result, September 6, 2016, was the date of my first chemo treatment. And I also met with a nutritionist on that day.

What have I learned up to this point?

First, ask a friend to accompany you to your medical meetings, particularly when dealing with a terminal diagnosis (even if your spouse is with you). A third party is not as emotionally invested as the family going through the crisis, and they tend to listen more keenly, ask more questions, and take better notes.

Second, in my melancholy state, for example, I forgot that I had done a scan a few days earlier, which would serve as a benchmark for chemo should I decide to move forward with treatment. Thankfully, Paulette, who was with me when the scan was done, remembered about it and asked the doctor what was the result of the scan. And hearing that the cancer had not spread to other organs, that was when I decided to move forward with chemo.

ANTICIPATING CHEMO REGIMENT

(Encouraged by the song below)

You may be down and feel like God has somehow forgotten
That you are faced with circumstances you can't get through
But now it seems that there's no way out and you're going under
God's proven time and time again; He'll take care of you

And He'll do it again; He'll do it again; If you'll just take a look
At where you are now; And where you've been
Well hasn't He always come through for
you; He's the same now as then
You may not know how; You may not
know when; But He'll do it again

God knows the things you're going through
and He knows how you're hurting
You see he knows just how you're heart has been broken in two
But He's the God of the stars, of the sun and
the sea; And He is your Father;
You see He can calm the storm; And He'll
find some way to fix it for you

Oh He's still God and He will not fail you; Oh
He's still God and He will not change
Know that He's God and He's fighting for you

ANGELLA DIXON-WATSON

Yes, just like Moses, just like Daniel; And just
like Shadrach and Meshach, Abednego

You may not know how; And you may not know when
You may not know how; You may not know when
But I know that He'll do it again
He'll do it again, again

Before I started chemo regiment, my friend Norma encouraged me to consult with a friend of hers in New York, who worked for years in the Oncology Department of one of the hospitals. I made the contact and am grateful that I did. Bottom line, the chat helped me to be less fearful of the journey ahead of me.

CHEMO REGIMENT

The oncologist gave me a treatment protocol of six months, which started Tuesday, September 6, 2016. I took chemo twenty-one days each month and had one week off.

- 2500 mg of Xeloda tablets taken daily at home
- 1000 mg of Gemzar infusion given weekly at Greenbaum Cancer Center, Baltimore
- 2000 mg of Xeloda (dosage changed from 2500 mg due to complications)

Remember that this is your body, so immediately report complications from the drugs you are taking (maybe dosage has to be changed).

On Tuesdays when I went to the Greenbaum Cancer Center, I was blessed to work with a supportive team. I was always anxious when it was time to do labs, although I had a portacath. Feel free to ask for the technician that you feel most comfortable with when doing labs and vitals, and that is what I started to do. And, here is why. On a Tuesday, my usual infusion day, my regular technicians Courtney, Trayonna or Tammy were unavailable. So, a person I never saw before came to take more labs (earlier that morning I had already done labs but it appears that there was an order to get more blood work). She had difficulty finding my portacath and I felt anxious after getting stuck many times without any success. And, I had a panic attack, fainted, and ended up in the emergency section and then was in the hospital for 2 days. I kept sharing with the staff that it was a panic attack but since my heart rate was so high and I had other health issues they decided to observe me.

Typical Day at the Cancer Center

- Register and wait in reception area until called to do vitals and lab.
- Before doing vitals, you are asked to both verify level of pain between 1 and 10 and give your name.
- Do vitals and labs, and it takes about one and a half hours for lab report to be back.
- Nurse gets report, and if lab report does not satisfy the benchmark for receiving chemo, you may not get treated, or infusion dosage may be adjusted for that session.
- Nurse orders medication from pharmacy; medication is made specifically for you. This may take another one and a half hours.
- Two pills are administered prior to infusion. They are to prevent nausea and infection.
- Medication is received from the pharmacy, and it is administered via IV. (Before it is administered, two nurses verified my name and date of birth. In my case, the infusion was for thirty minutes.)

I recall that on more than one occasion, my white blood cells count was below the benchmark and it was a cause of great concern. Eventually, however, the drug was given but dosage was adjusted to a lesser amount. Thankfully, my first experience having low white blood cells count happened when my friend Uva, a nurse, accompanied me to treatment. I was tearful and confused during the low white blood cells count dialogue between the nurse and myself. I kept saying to Uva what are they saying to me — what is happening — she kept me calm; was very careful with her words and reassured me that everything would be okay. So, when the scenario of "low white blood cells count" happened again, I felt confident that I would make it through.

While getting the infusion, I often listened to songs on my phone and one in particular was:

> In Shady Green Pastures, So rich and so FREE
> God Leads his dear children along
> Some through the water, Some through the flood
> Some through the valley but all through the blood

I observed that a nurse administering my liquid chemo (Gemzar) often wore two gloves and two gowns. On one occasion, I asked why and she said "that she did not want to accidentally let the drug touch her." It was another reality check for me that the drug was destroying good and bad cells. And, that only God could deliver me from this illness.

> The Lord sent his word, and healed them And delivered them from their destruction He sent his word to heal them and preserve their life (Ps. 107:20, Moffat)

Trips to Baltimore for liquid infusion of chemo treatment was once weekly and we tapped into offers from friends and family who wanted to accompany me. Ira wanted to take me every time, but I wanted to give him a break. He never wavered in his support during the entire 7-1/2 months of chemo and radiation treatments. I am blessed to have him in my life.

My Side Effects

(God spared me from about 95% of typical side effects)

- Extreme sensitivity in palm of the hands (easier to use plastic utensils instead of metal)
- Extreme sensitivity in sole of feet (felt like prickles when walking)
- Sensitivity at the tip of my fingers
- Food taste changes
- Food smells bothersome
- Some tiredness
- Some hair thinning after about 5 months
- Some nausea (when doing both chemo and radiation)
- Discoloration of nails and face

What is neutropenia?

Neutropenia is the condition of not having enough white blood cells to fight infection. As a result, I was encouraged to be on the alert if I got a fever of 100.4 or greater. I should not take any aids to relieve it but go directly to the hospital and show the staff my alert card. The card shows type of cancer and drugs I am taking. It was also wise to travel with a mask to prevent infections when going to public places.

On days when I completed chemo and may not be experiencing many side effects, oh, how I wished my friend, Jenny J, was still living next door to bring me some Trini roti and bake and that would save me a trip to the Roti shop in Langley park.

Chemo and a Changed Mind-Set

When going through a life-threatening illness, your mind-set must be positive. I am a human being, and yes, there were days of tears and concerns. The devil whispered all kinds of negatives in my ears, and you have to fight back with the word of God and imagine yourself healed—not being healed. Once again, *healed!*

As an encouragement to others, remember that when a pebble is thrown in a body of water, ripples are seen on the surface. However, the living creatures underneath the surface are not disturbed. So, keep hidden in our hearts the words of God, and repeating them gives you strength.

> Behold, I give you the authority to trample on serpents and scorpions, and over all the power of the enemy, and nothing shall by any means hurt you. (Luke 10:19)

> The thief does not come except to steal, and to kill And to destroy I have come that you may have life, And that you have it more abundantly. (John 10:10)

> The tongue has power of life and death. The talkative must take the consequences (Prov. 18:21, Moffat)

GIFT OF ANOTHER BREATH

Once I decided to move ahead with my treatment, I refused to allow the enemy to control my mind. So, when doubts popped up and sometimes they did, I tried not to linger in that space. I reminded myself of Mrs. Osteen's miraculous healing and I also went to the "word."

I spoke positively over my life daily. According to scriptures, the world came into being through words. Genesis 1:3 and God said, "Let there be …"

> So I say to you, ask, and it will be given to you; seek
> and you will find; knock and it will be opened to you.
> (Luke 11:9)

As a result, I changed my speech pattern: from "I am going to take this poison, referring to the chemo," I said instead, "This is my healing medicine."

Therefore I say to you, whatsoever you ask When you pray, believe that you receive them And you will have them (Mark 11:24)

At home, I walked around and talked loudly. This is what I said:

> Satan, you tried to take me out silently
> But God stopped you
> He made me itch and scratch so severely
> And made me so jaundiced I
> could not ignore the signs
> And I sought medical attention
> You lost!

Daily Juicing Protocol

(While doing chemo)

Morning smoothie

I prepared a smoothie made of kale, spinach, watercress, radish, fennel, asparagus, brussel sprouts, moringa, wheatgrass, aloe vera, ginger, and any other greens I had. The chaser was coconut water. I chose two items from the list (watercress being the base and fresh ginger).

Lunch smoothie

I prepared a fruit drink using at least two different fruits (apple, cantaloupe, watermelon, berries or any other fruit). My base was fresh pineapple and ginger.

Dinner smoothie

I used carrot as the base with one other item, such as fennel, beets, celery, turmeric, chia or flaxseed for omega 3, mixed nuts. The chaser was unsweetened almond milk.

There are other purchases I made at the organic store that I used on an ad hoc basis. If you can't do juicing, do what you can. You may consider going to organic shops or go down the organic aisle of your local supermarkets, and you may find items that can nourish your body; for example, powdered organic super green food and organic protein drinks.

I also included soups made from all types of beans and peas.

The key is to *overdose* on nutrition.

In addition to the above, I drank at least 32–48 ounces of water daily, and it should have been more due to the daily chemo intake. Oftentimes, I used water that was alkaline. And I sometimes added fresh lemon to regular bottled water.

I stayed away from a meat-based diet 99 percent of the time. I was *not* perfect. The national dish of Jamaica is ackee and codfish. And I could not see myself having ackee without the codfish. Nor, go by Mitchie and Percy for Thanksgiving dinner and not have a taste of Jamaican-style jerk chicken and escovitched fish, which is a well-seasoned fish made with hot peppers, onions, and other spices.

Honestly, during my small indulgence at Thanksgiving, I could hear my friend Beverly's voice in my head restating the dangers of non-plant-based diet. And I agree with her. She is my plant-based "dietary conscience." I follow a dietary path that is about 99 percent plant based.

Chemo-Free Weeks

In addition to the chemo regiment previously shared, during the week that I did not do chemo (tablets or liquid), I drank different herb teas, and here are a few examples: guinea hen, moringa, soursop, pomegranate, red clover, Flor Essence (Essiac), cinnamon, ginger, and green tea. I also took multivitamins.

CANCER FREE

Wednesday, February 22, 2017

On Valentine's Day, after my usual chemo infusion at the Greenbaum Cancer Center, first floor, I went to Radiation Oncology on the lower level of the hospital and did a scan. This scan would determine if chemo for the last six months was a success and to establish the protocol for radiation treatment. On our way home from the hospital, Paulette (who accompanied me on this trip for both chemo and radiation treatments) and I stopped at Negril restaurant in Laurel to treat ourselves to a nice island cuisine before heading home to hang out with our spouses. Within minutes after ordering, our friend Heather came through the door to see her staff. The three of us sat together and what would have normally been a 45 minutes "eat in" ended up being over 3 hours chit chatting, laughing and catching up on life! It was refreshing.

On the morning of Wednesday, February 22, I was given the results of the scan, and I was declared *cancer free*! The chemo taken over the last six months worked. There were *no* signs of cancer in my body. This *was* a miracle. Prayers worked.

I was also told that I was one of 15 percent of patients with pancreatic cancer who *even* made it to surgery!

Based on the above scan results, the protocol was established to start daily radiation. From what I understood, radiation would focus on the area where the cancer was found to prevent it from returning.

> Your sickness will leave and not come back again.
> What do you conspire against the LORD? He will

make an utter end of it. Affliction will not rise up a second time. (Nah. 1:9)

It is God's will for you to be healed. And behold, a leper came and worshipped Him, saying, "Lord, if You are willing, You can make me clean." Then Jesus put out His hand and touched him, saying, "I am willing; be cleansed." Immediately his leprosy was cleansed. (Matt. 8:2–3)

Radiation and Continued Chemo

Wednesday, February 22

Although I was already declared cancer free, my heart sank when I was informed that the protocol was for me to continue with chemo while doing radiation. I had just completed six months of a rigorous chemo schedule, and I was unsure that my body could take both chemo and radiation at the same time.

I started daily radiation treatment on Monday, February 27, 2017, for five and a half weeks (no treatment on weekends).

I was so blessed to have a supportive radiation oncology team starting from the receptionists. On one occasion, while waiting to meet with my Radiation Oncology doctor, Nurse William greeted me with a big ear to ear smile and said "hello star." He and I bursted out laughing and during this exchange my spirit screamed thankfulness to God for showing his ongoing healing mercy towards me. In the Radiation Oncology section, patients entered through the double front doors and into the inner radiation reception area. You go to a room which had a locker and you change clothing by putting on a gown and wait to be called to go on the machine. Before going on the machine you are asked to give your name and date of birth.

In the radiation room, I had my own headrest molded just for me to make me comfortable. I had four markers on my body, one on each side and two on my stomach. I held on to two bars behind my head while a three-pronged machine circled my body, and this position was tiring at times. The lasers earmarked where the markers were located on my body. The machine stopped and started a few times, and the process took about fifteen to twenty minutes.

Sometimes music was playing in the room, and, I heard the following song: "Let the Church Say Amen."

In addition to radiation, I continued to take 2000 mg of Xeloda chemo tablets daily at home. I did not take Xeloda on weekends since radiation was not administered.

On one of my visits for radiation, I was told that I *was* one of 10 percent who is successfully making it through radiation and chemotherapy.

This regiment made me lethargic, and with prayers, I successfully completed this protocol on Tuesday, April 4.

On my final day of radiation, I received a certificate from Radiation Oncology acknowledging that I successfully completed the regiment. At this hospital, when one completes radiation, there is a victory bell in the reception hall that one can ring if they so desire. I did not ring the bell, didn't want to bring too much attention to myself!

> I will bless the LORD at all times; his praise shall continually be in my mouth. My soul shall make her boast in the LORD: the humble shall hear thereof, and be glad. O magnify the LORD with me, and let us exalt his name together. I sought the LORD, and he heard me, and delivered me from all my fears. (Ps. 34: 1–4)

ENCOURAGEMENTS IN DIFFERENT WAYS

I read healing scriptures. I bought CDs filled with healing songs and my friend Mitchie gave me CDs filled with praise and worship songs. I also purchased two identical CDs called *Healing Scriptures*, narrated by Kenneth Copeland. I figured that I may give away the extra copy to someone at the cancer center.

Planting of Seeds

> Sow your seed in the morning, and do not stop working until the evening for you do not know which activity will succeed whether this one or that one, or whether both will prosper equally. (Eccles. 11:6, Moffat version)

The opportunity came to give away the extra copy of the *Healing Scriptures* CD when a friend's wife had surgery and was going to start radiation.

Also, in the oncology reception areas, they have different types of magazines, and not all on health. So oftentimes, I added my magazines *Visitor* and *Adventist World*.

On my last day of radiation and chemo treatments (Tuesday, April 4), I gave away to a fellow radiation patient my only copy of *Healing Scriptures* CD. And within the same week, Thursday to be exact, the mailman dropped off a package, and I wondered who this was coming from. When I opened the package, it was filled with Kenneth Copeland Ministries (KCM) series on healing. And the

CD I gave away on Tuesday was replaced on Thursday. The invoice showed zero balance!

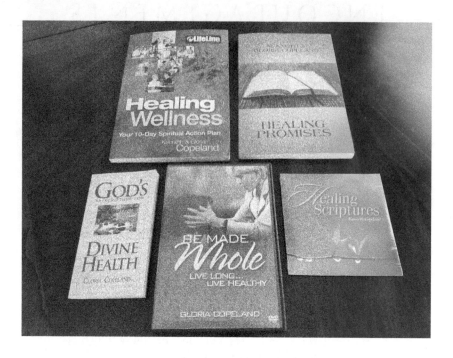

"Healing"

Ira was a longtime friend of Kenneth and Gloria Copeland's. He had already shared with KCM about my health situation, and they prayed for me and blessed us in many other ways beyond prayer. The blessings and gifts received from KCM was a stark reminder of God's goodness and faithfulness to his people.

Allow me to provide a historical perspective. From 1982 to 1986, Ira had the distinct honor and privilege of ministering onstage with Kenneth Copeland all over the world. As a staff musician, music producer, singer, and songwriter with the ministry, Ira ministered with Kenneth and Gloria from the Sydney Opera House in Australia to Birmingham, England, and beyond.

During this phase of Ira's life with KCM, he learned valuable lessons about relying on God and believing the Word. So when my illness occurred, he knew that he had to go to the Rock of our salvation, which is God. "I have not forgotten you my son, and because you have set your love upon me, you shall call upon me and I will answer."

So Ira called on Him, and He answered and gave him strength to be a faithful caretaker to me!

> I urge you, brothers and sisters, by our Lord Jesus Christ and by the love of the Spirit, to join me in my struggle by praying to God for me. (Rom. 15:30)
>
> As you help us by your prayers. Then many will give thanks on our behalf for the gracious favor granted us in answer to the prayers of many. (2 Cor. 1:11)

Protocol after Chemo and Radiation Were Completed

Apart from requesting to be fully healed, my other big wish was that I would not be placed on maintenance chemo drugs after treatment protocol was over. God is faithful and He granted my requests. In addition, my Oncologist encouraged me to keep doing what I had been doing? What was I doing?

I Believed in God for My Healing

> Therefore I say to you
> Whatsoever things you ask when you pray
> Believe that you receive them and you will have them (Mark 11:24)
>
> But he was wounded for our transgressions
> He was bruised for our inequities
> The chastisement of our peace was on him
> And with His stripes I am healed (Isaiah 53:5)
>
> If you remain in me and my words remain in you,
> Then ask whatever you like and you shall
> have it (John 15: 7, Moffat version)

There is a song that goes,

ANGELLA DIXON-WATSON

Mercy rewrote my life
Mercy rewrote my life
I could have fallen my soul cast down
But mercy rewrote my life

My mistakes God turned into miracles
And all of my tears He turned into Joy
Then my past was forgiven and my new name it was written
When mercy rewrote my life

MOVING FORWARD

Quiet Celebration

Now the new week had begun, and I was walking around at home dazed. I kept saying to myself, *Am I really not getting dressed to go to Baltimore for the daily or weekly treatments I had been going to for seven and a half months?* Wow, treatment is really over, and God has granted my wish for healing!

And here is one more good news! I did not lose more weight during treatment. Before I started on the journey, I was 164 pounds. Then by the time I started chemo, I was 127.4 pounds; and now at the end of my journey, I am at 140 pounds. I recall that on one of Marva's visits, she said to me, "Are you gaining weight?" I laughed and cheerfully said yes.

> God is for you. For all the promises of God in Him are
> Yes, and in Him Amen, to the glory of God through
> us. (2 Cor. 1:20)

God will fulfill the number of my days. He has the final say. You have granted me life and loving kindness; And Your care has preserved my spirit. Job 10:12

The new treatment protocol is for me to meet with both the oncologist and radiation oncologist once every three months for two years. And gradually, the visits would be spread out over a longer period of time. During this time also, CT scans and lab tests would be administered.

Mental Dialogue

Again, I am human and not perfect.

Here comes the enemy's whispers. Okay, you are cancer free, so what are you going to do with the hundred chemo tablets you have left? Might as well keep them because, you never know—you may need them again.

It took me about two weeks to finally dispose of the tablets.

> Do not give the devil a foothold. (Eph. 4:27)

I asked God to give me strength not to believe the enemy's lies. I asked Him to give me strength to believe in His words on complete healing. I kept repeating Nahum 1:9 "He will make a full end; affliction shall not rise up the second time."

> I will bless the LORD at all times: his praise shall continually be in my mouth. (Ps. 34:1)

> I sought the LORD, and he heard me, and delivered me from all my fears. The angel of the LORD encamps round about them that fear him, and delivers them. *(Ps. 34:4, 34:7)*

> *God is our refuge and strength, a very present help in trouble.* (Ps. 46:1)

DIET

I will continue on the dietary path I embarked on during this journey and will research ways to make improvements. I will also keep closely in touch with my "plant based dietary" friends Beverly, Claudette and the Drakes for continued encouragement down this path.

> The LORD will guide you always; he will satisfy your needs in a sun-scorched land and will strengthen your frame. You will be like a well-watered garden, like a spring whose waters never fail. (Isa. 58:11)

CONTINUING ACTIVITIES

Meditation, socializing, travel, and exercise.

In order to have a more balanced life, I will adopt meditation as a form of stress relief by praying, reading and listening to varying kinds of music. Stress that is left unchecked can contribute to health problems.

Socialization: I am energized when I am around people. My plan is to get more involved in community based humanitarian projects and be a face of inspiration and hope.

Travel: I plan to do more international traveling to learn more of different cultures and lifestyles. I enjoy chit chatting with natives and visitors on the beaches of my hometown, Montego Bay, Jamaica.

Exercise: Walking and dancing to different genres of music are forms of exercises I enjoy. When I go for walks, I leave my phone at home and just enjoy the beauty of creation without being interrupted.

REMEMBRANCE

My deliverance is humbling. And I ask God to help me never to forget his grace and mercy. I will remember the story of the Potter and the clay. I recall also that when Joshua and the children of Israel crossed the river Jordan, stones were placed in the river for a purpose, and instructions were given:

> Then Joshua said to the Israelites, "In the future your children will ask, 'What do these stones mean?' Then you can tell them, 'This is where the Israelites crossed the Jordan on dry ground.'
>
> For the LORD your God dried up the river right before your eyes, and he kept it dry until you were all across, just as he did at the Red Sea when he dried it up until we had all crossed over. He did this so all the nations of the earth might know that the LORD's hand is powerful, and so you might fear the LORD your God forever." (Josh. 4: 21–24)

What is my takeaway from this journey?

1. Follow your heart and choose the health and healing paths that are best for you. Listen to your heart more than to your mind. Our minds tend to lead us down analytical paths. *"Above all else, guard your heart, for everything you do flows from it"* (Prov. 4:23).

2. Be prepared to live with the consequences of your decision.

3. Trust God and have faith. Here is a simple formula: praise builds faith.

4. Defeat the spirit of fear by pulling on the words of God hidden in your heart. Remember that the spirits we do not see are more real than the world we see. *"For God has not given us a spirit of fear but of power, and of love and of a sound mind"* (2 Tim. 1:7).

5. During moments of sadness, have a Bible verse or a song that you can immediately repeat in the *"blink of an eye."*

6. Open your mouths and praise God. Use praise as a defense mechanism, and the enemy will flee. *"He put a new song in my mouth, a hymn of praise to our God. Many will see and fear the LORD and put their trust in him"* (Ps. 40:3). Exercising this mode of operation brings a special kind of energy to your mind, body, and soul.

7. Be thankful. Develop a spirit of gratitude. Being grateful energizes our soul and contributes to healing.

HEALING SCRIPTURES

Here are a few scriptures that Gilbert and Christopher had written out for me when they visited.

Jeremiah 32:27

Behold, I am the Lord, the God of all flesh. Is there anything too hard for me?

Mark 11:24

Therefore I say to you, whatever things you ask when you pray, believe that you receive them, and you will have them.

James 1:6

But let him ask in faith, with no doubting, for he who doubts is like a wave of the sea driven and tossed by the sea.

Luke 11:9

So I say to you, ask, and it will be given to you; seek and you will find; knock and it will be opened to you.

ADDITIONAL COMFORTING SCRIPTURES

John 15:7

If ye abide in me, and my words abide in you, ye shall ask what ye will, and it shall be done unto you.

Psalms 107:20
The Lord sent his words and heals them and delivered them from their destruction.

Romans 10:17

So then faith cometh by hearing and hearing by the word of God

Psalms 105:37

He brought them forth also with silver and gold and there was not one feeble person among their tribes

Mathew 21:14

And the blind and the lame came to him in the temple; and he healed them

Isaiah 41:10

So do not fear, for I am with you; do not be dismayed, for I am your God. I will strengthen you and help you; I will uphold you with my righteous right hand

John 3:2

Beloved, I wish above all things that thou may prosper and be in health, even as thy soul prospers.

Mark 5:34

He said to her, "Daughter, your faith has healed you. Go in peace and be freed from your suffering."

    This journal will always serve as a reminder to me that God is faithful. Expectancy, waiting and believing are breeding grounds for miracles and my positive prognosis of this miracle claims "God" as my physician and healer. Let's celebrate the abundance of favors God has granted us second by second through the daily "Gift of Another Breath." My hope is that my story, scriptures and songs will bless my family and you.

ACKNOWLEDGMENTS

Phone and text visitors and prayer groups

The list is extensive. You know who you are, and I am forever grateful.

To my unofficially adopted brothers

Clinton, Dean, Basil, Vilroy, Clive, Archie and Rob, who kept my spirit up by sending me cheerful emojis, and island jokes via texting.

A special thanks to Raquel-Ann's adopted godmother, Arlene, and the staff at Brandon House (ARC of Prince Georges County) for being supportive in many ways. In addition, I also thank former manager Jackie. Ms. Joyce, also previously of the ARC, sent me cards practically every month. Here are the words from one of the cards, which had a bright yellow background, image of the sun, red roses and a red bird with yellow stripes, yellow beak and it was sitting on a tree limb: "I Care and thought this might be a good time to remind you. Sending smiles and good wishes."

Family members, In-laws and friends and unknown persons

Thank you for your prayers, gifts, cuisines, bouquets, cards, home checks, text and phone calls.

Home Visitors

Salome, Gwen, Norma, Andrea, Beverly; Mitchie and Percy; Joy, Stella, Gem; Vickie and Mary; Jenny and Oliver; Moyna and Michael; Sandy, Jean and Christiana; Uva and Frank; Gilbert and Christopher; Bertram and Cavel; Frazier family; Evan and Tia; Winsome and Trudy; Grace, Ucley and Angelia; Danny and Vinette; Ervin, Claude and Sheldon; Faye and Alex; Donna-Marie and Winston; Esther, Nicole and Pansy; Winsome and Florence; Rachel and Carmen (in-laws).

Tia was the youngest of my visitors and a high school student. It was refreshing to see how articulate and dedicated she was in her studies. Her aim is to make a valuable contribution to society in the areas of science and robotics. While conversing with her, I learned that her mom, Evan, taught her faith principles. And, I was encouraged to hold on to my faith and to believe in healing miracles.

GIFT OF ANOTHER BREATH

To the medical team and their staff

H. Richard Alexander, Jr., MD
Professor and Associate Chairman for Clinical Research
Division of General and Oncologic Surgery
University of Maryland, Baltimore

Yixing Jiang, MD, PhD
Associate Professor of Medicine
Director, GI Medical Oncology
University of Maryland, Baltimore

William F. Regine, MD, FACRO
Isadore and Fannie Schneider Foxman Chair and Professor of Radiation Oncology
Executive Director, Maryland Proton Treatment Center (MPTC)
Department of Radiation Oncology
University of Maryland, Baltimore

Raymond E. Kim, MD
Department of Gastroenterology
University of Maryland, Baltimore

Padmaja Udapi, MD
Primary Care Physician
Diplomate of the American Board of Internal Medicine
Infectious Disease and Internal Medicine

Eileen R. Erskine, CRNP
Capital Digestive Care

Martha Francis, CRNP
Department of Radiation Oncology
University of Maryland, Baltimore

Kim Alumbaugh, RN, CCM
Conifer Health Solutions

ENCOURAGEMENTS

I initially started journaling on an ad hoc basis with the intention to jot down just enough information so that our grandchildren Cierra and Chase could know a little more about "Nana's" health journey and also her ancestry for the benefit of future generations.

In the process of doing limited journaling, my childhood friend, Esther Kerr, encouraged me to seriously consider writing my story. I was unsure if I wanted to publicly share my journey. However, after much prodding from her, I became serious. And, about six months after I started, I shared with friends that I was journaling, and I received more encouragements. Ira was also a great source of support. And, not realizing it, the journal was finished on Thursday, July 27 —exactly one year after I was told, "You have pancreatic cancer." I do not believe in coincidences!

Why did I choose Covenant publishers? About two years ago I felt that I needed a closer relationship with God. So, I randomly opened my bible and the following scripture popped up which I memorized and used as my "go to" when feeling disconnected.: "Yet I will remember the covenant I made with you in the days of your youth, and I will establish an everlasting covenant with you." Ezekiel 16:60.

Well, fast forward to now. In July, I decided to research a publisher I heard about on TV and radio so I googled their information and was impressed. Then, I listened intently to my spirit and I heard the whisper of a small voice saying to me -- would they understand the meanings of your biblical references and songs? My spirit said

No. I continued my google search looking for a christian publisher and then I came up on Covenant books and then I said "Yes" This in my opinion is one of the fulfillments of Eze. 16:60.

Listening to our inner spirit is very important. My friend, Marva, is a listening advocate and founder of "I love to Listen Day" celebrated on May 16th each year, which is the premier international listening day. She strongly believes in the biblical importance "Everyone should be quick to listen, slow to speak" James 1:19 and also " Listen to counsel and receive instruction, that you may be wise in your latter days." —*Proverbs 19:20.*

Nurturing Praise and Worship Songs That Ministered to My Soul

LARGER THAN LIFE

Before the Heavens
Far Beyond the Stars
Before the Milky Way
And Moon Beams on Mars
And Before I was a Gleam in My Mother's Eyes

You were Larger, Larger Than Life
You Are Larger, Greater Than Life

Ocean of Tears Fell
Down My Tear Stained Face
When I Heard you say Redeemed I Realized

You Are Larger, Larger Than Life
You Are Larger, Greater Than Life

(Bridge)
Palm Trees In Paradise Bow Down To You
Oh how the Wind and Waves Obey and Applaud you

(Words and music by Ira Watson)

BLESSED ASSURANCE

1. Blessed assurance, Jesus is mine!
Oh, what a foretaste of glory divine!
Heir of salvation, purchase of God,
Born of His Spirit, washed in His blood.

o *Refrain*
This is my story, this is my song,
Praising my Savior all the day long;
This is my story, this is my song,
Praising my Savior all the day long.
o

2. Perfect submission, perfect delight,
Visions of rapture now burst on my sight;
Angels, descending, bring from above
Echoes of mercy, whispers of love.

3. Perfect submission, all is at rest,
I in my Savior am happy and blest,
Watching and waiting, looking above,
Filled with His goodness, lost in His love.

HEALING

Healing is Here, Healing is Here
And I receive it; Healing is here, Healing is here
I receive it
I lift my head to the heavens; I lift my eyes to where my
Help comes from
I look to you my rock my healer, I trust in you

Sickness can't stay any longer…
Your perfect love is casting out fear; You are the God of all power
And it's your will that my life be healed

KEEP ME SAFE UNTIL THE STORM PASSES BY

In the dark of the midnight have I oft hid my face
While the storm howls above me, and there's no hiding place
'Mid the crash of the thunder, Precious Lord, hear my cry
Keep me safe till the storm passes by

Till the storm passes over, till the thunder sounds no more
Till the clouds roll forever from the sky
Hold me fast, let me stand in the hollow of Thy hand
Keep me safe till the storm passes by

HEALING IN THIS HOUSE

There is healing in this house - healing in this house
Manifested peace to all
Troubled hearts with healing balm.

There is healing in this house.
Restoration in this place.

There is mercy there is grace
Though you're heavy laden come.
Bring your burdens one by one.
Leave them here where they belong.
There is healing in this house.

WELCOME HOLY SPIRIT

Be here with your presence
Fill me with your power
Live inside of me

You're the living water
Never drying fountain
Comforter and counselor
Take complete control

PRECIOUS LORD, TAKE MY HAND

Precious Lord, take my hand; Lead me on, let me stand
I'm tired, I'm weak, I'm lone
Through the storm, through the night; Lead me on to the light
Take my hand precious Lord, lead me home

When my way grows drear, precious Lord linger near
When my light is almost gone; Hear my cry, hear my call

Hold my hand lest I fall
Take my hand precious Lord, lead me home

HOLY SPIRIT

Hover o'er me, Holy Spirit,
Bathe my trembling heart and brow;
Fill me with Thy hallowed presence,
Come, O come and fill me now.
Fill me now, fill me now,
Jesus, come and fill me now;
Fill me with Thy hallowed presence,
Come, O come, and fill me now.

SHELTER FROM THE STORM

The Lord's our Rock, in Him we hide,
A Shelter in the time of storm;
Secure whatever ill betide,
A Shelter in the time of storm.
Oh, Jesus is a Rock in a weary land,
A weary land, a weary land;
Oh, Jesus is a Rock in a weary land,
A Shelter in the time of storm.

HOW GREAT THOU ART

Oh Lord my God
When I in awesome wonder
Consider all the worlds
Thy hands have made
I see the stars
I hear the rolling thunder
Thy power throughout
The universe displayed

Then sings my soul
My Savior, God, to Thee
How great thou art
How great thou art

THANK YOU

Oh Lord, I thank you, thank you, thank you
Oh Lord, I thank you, thank you, thank you
I just thank you for the joy in my heart.
Oh Lord, I thank you,
I really thank you,
I just thank you for the joy in my heart.

When I was lost, Lord, you found me,
When I was hungry, Lord, you fed me,
When I was sick, Lord, you healed me
And I will thank you all the days of my Life.

Welcome Holy spirit
We are in his presence
Fill us with your power
Live inside of me

NO SECRET WHAT GOD CAN DO

The chimes of time ring out the news, another day is through
Someone slipped and fell, was that someone you?
You may have longed for added strength your courage to renew
Do not be disheartened, I have news for you

It is no secret what God can do
What he's done for others he'll do for you
With arms wide open, he'll pardon you
It is no secret what God can do

WHEN WE ALL GET TO HEAVEN

Sing the wondrous love of Jesus,
Sing His mercy and His grace;
In the mansions bright and blessed
He'll prepare for us a place.
When we all get to heaven,
What a day of rejoicing that will be!
When we all see Jesus,
We'll sing and shout the victory!

YOUR GRACE AND MERCY

Your grace and mercy brought me through
I'm living this moment because of You
I want to thank You, and praise You too
Your grace and mercy brought me through

Thank You, for saving a sinner like me
To tell the world salvation is free
There were times when I just didn't do right
But You watched over me
All day and night

SO YOU WOULD KNOW

How many times must I prove how much I love you?
How many times, must my love for you I show?
And how many times must I rescue you from trouble?
For you to know just how much I love you.
Chorus
Didn't I wake you up this morning,
You were clothed in your right mind
And didn't you walk right in your closet,
Each step right in time.
When you were weak on life's journey,
Didn't my angels carry you?
So you would know
So you would know
So you would know just how much I love you.
How many days must I build a fence around you?
And how many nights must I wipe all yours tears away?
And how many storms must I bring you safely through?
For you to know how much I love you.
Chorus
Didn't I put food on your table,
When your bills were all past due?

And when the pain was bad in your body,
Didn't I send healing right to you?

When you were lost in sin and sorrow,
Well, I died just to set you free
So you would know
So you would know
So you would know just how much I really love you.

THE BLOOD WILL NEVER LOSE ITS POWER

The blood that Jesus shed for me,
Way back on Calvary;
The blood that gives me strength

From day to day,
It will never lose its power.

It reaches to the highest mountain,
It flows to the lowest valley;
The blood that gives me strength
From day to day,
It will never lose its power.

It soothes my doubts and calms my fears,
And it dries all my tears;
The blood that gives me strength
From day to day,
It will never lose its power.

PUT YOUR HAND

Put your hand in the hand of the man who stilled the water
Put your hand in the hand of the man who calmed the sea
Take a look at yourself and you can look at others diff'rently
Put your hand in the hand of the man from Galilee

BALM IN GILEAD

Sometimes I feel discouraged and think my work's in vain,
But then the Holy Spirit revives my soul again.

There is a balm in Gilead to make the wounded whole;
There is a balm in Gilead to heal the sin sick soul.
Don't ever feel discouraged, for Jesus is your friend;
And if you lack for knowledge, He'll never refuse to lend.
There is a balm in Gilead to make the wounded whole;
There is a balm in Gilead to heal the sin sick soul

JESUS IS THE LIGHTHOUSE

There's a lighthouse on the hillside
That overlooks life's sea
When I'm tossed it sends out
A light that I might see
And the light that shines in darkness
Now will safely lead me home
If it wasn't for the lighthouse
My ship would be no more

And I thank God for the lighthouse
I owe my life to Him
Jesus is the lighthouse
And from the rocks of sin
He has shown the light around me
That I mighty clearly see
If it wasn't for the lighthouse
Tell me: where would this ship be?

WASH AWAY SINS

What can wash away my sin?
Nothing but the blood of Jesus;
What can make me whole again?
Nothing but the blood of Jesus.

Oh! Precious is the flow
That makes me white as snow;
No other fount I know,
Nothing but the blood of Jesus

PEACE IN THE MIDST OF THE STORM

When the world that I've been
Living in collapses at my feet
And when my life is all tattered and torn
Though I'm wind-swept, I've been battered
I'm gonna cling unto His cross
I'll find peace in the midst of the storm

There is peace in the midst of the storm-tossed life
There is an Anchor, there is a rock to build my faith upon
Jesus Christ is my vessel so I fear no alarm
He gives me peace in the midst of the storm

DOUBTS ARE SETTLED

But it's real, it's real;
Oh, I know it's real;
Praise God, the doubts are settled,
For I know, I know it's real!
But at last I tired of living such a life of fear and doubt,
For I wanted God to give me something I would know about,
So the truth would make me happy and
the light would clearly shine,
And the Spirit give assurance that I'm His and He is mine.

WASHED MY EYES WITH TEARS

He washed my eyes with tears that I might see,
The broken heart I had was good for me;
He tore it all apart and looked inside,
He found it full of fear and foolish pride.
He swept away the things that made me blind
And then I saw the clouds were silver lined;
And now I understand 'twas best for me
He washed my eyes with tears that I might see.

He washed my eyes with tears that I might see
The glory of Himself revealed to me;
I did not know that He had wounded hands
I saw the blood He spilt upon the sands.
I saw the marks of shame and wept and cried;
He was my substitute for me He died;
And now I'm glad He came so tenderly;
And washed my eyes with tears that I might see.

LILY OF THE VALLEY

I have found a friend in Jesus, He's ev'rything to me,
He's the fairest of ten thousand to my soul;
The Lily of the Valley, in Him alone I see
All I need to cleanse and make me fully whole:
In sorrow He's my comfort, in trouble He's my stay;
He tells me ev'ry care on Him to roll;
He's the Lily of the Valley, the Bright and Morning Star,
He's the fairest of ten thousand to my soul.

STORM PASSES BY

Keep me save till the storm passes by
In the dark of the midnight, Have I oft hid my face;
While the storm howls above me,
And there's no hiding place;
'Mid the crash of the thunder, Precious Lord, hear my cry;
"Keep me safe 'til the storm passes by."

'Til the storm passes over,
'Til the thunder sounds no more; 'Til the
clouds roll forever from the sky,
Hold me fast, let me stand, In the hollow of Thy hand;
Keep me safe 'til the storm passes by.

Many times Satan whispers,
"There is no need to try; For there's no end of sorrow,
There's no hope by and by";
But I know Thou art with me, And tomorrow I'll rise;
Where the storms never darken the skies.

'Til the storm passes over,
'Til the thunder sounds no more; 'Til the
clouds roll forever from the sky,
Hold me fast, let me stand,
In the hollow of Thy hand; Keep me safe 'til the storm passes by.

When the long night has ended,
And the storms come no more, Let me stand in Thy presence.
On that bright, peaceful shore.
In that land where the tempest; Never comes, Lord may I
Dwell with Thee when the storm passes by.

'Til the storm passes over,
'Til the thunder sounds no more; 'Til the
clouds roll forever from the sky,
Hold me fast, let me stand,
In the hollow of Thy hand; Keep me safe 'til the storm passes by.

Hold me fast, Let me stand, In the hollow of Thy hand;
Keep me safe 'til the storm passes by.

I'VE GOT TO PRAISE HIM

When I think about what the Lord has done
When I think about where He's brought me from
When I think about all He's given me
When I think about the man who gave me victory
I can't help myself; I've got to praise Him

HEALING WATERS

Where the healing waters flow
Where there is peace and rest and love

Oh, the joy of sins forgiv'n,
Oh, the bliss the blood-wash'd know, Oh, the peace akin to heav'n,
Where the healing waters flow.

Chorus
Where the healing waters flow,
Where the joys celestial glow;
Oh, there's peace and rest and love,
Where the healing waters flow.

Now with Jesus crucified,
At His feet I'm resting low; Let me evermore abide
Where the healing waters flow.

Oh, this precious perfect love!
How it keeps the heart aglow; Streaming from the fount above,
Where the healing waters flow.

Oh, to lean on Jesus' breast,
While the tempests come and go! Here is blessed peace and rest,
Where the healing waters flow.

Cleans'd from ev'ry sin and stain,
Whiter than the driven snow, Now I sing my sweet refrain,
Where the healing waters flow

LEANING ON THE EVERLASTING ARMS

What a fellowship, what a joy divine,
Leaning on the everlasting arms;
What a blessedness, what a peace is mine,
Leaning on the everlasting arms.

Leaning, leaning,
Safe and secure from all alarms;
Leaning, leaning,
Leaning on the everlasting arms.

HE WILL CARRY ME

There is no problem too big
God cannot solve it
There is no mountain too tall
God cannot move it
There is no storm too dark
God cannot calm it
There is no sorrow too deep
He cannot soothe it
Oh, if He carried the weight of the world upon His shoulders
Oh, I know my brother that He will carry you
Oh, if He carried the weight of the world upon His shoulders
Oh, I know my sister that He will carry you
I know my brother and I know my sister that Jesus will carry you

HE RESCUED ME

On the stormy sea of sin I was sinking
Never to rise again
The wind and the rains 'round me crashing
Had battered and torn me within

But He rescued me, Jesus rescued me
From the cold dark waters of sin's troubled sea
He rescued me, new life I can see
Jesus reached down in love
And He rescued me.

I could feel death's arm around me
As I struggled for my life
I could see his angel waiting to claim me for his prize
In my hour of desperation I almost lost my mind
But somehow I cried to Jesus
And He saved me just in time.

DON'T BE DISCOURAGED

Don't be discouraged
Joy comes in the morning
Know that God is nigh
Stand still and look up
God is going to show up
He is standing by

There's healing for your sorrow
Healing for your pain
Healing for your spirit
There's shelter from the rain
Lord send the healing
For this we know
There is a balm in Gilead
For there's a balm in Gilead
There is a balm in Gilead
To heal the soul

Richard Smallwood

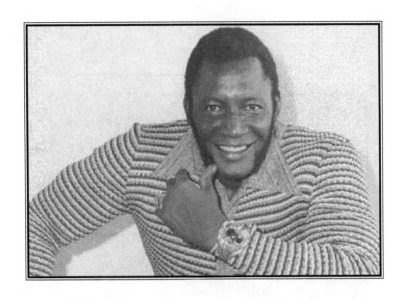

"Dorel"
Father

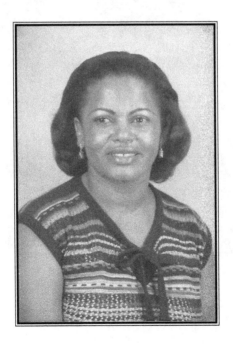

"Ms. Babs"
Mother

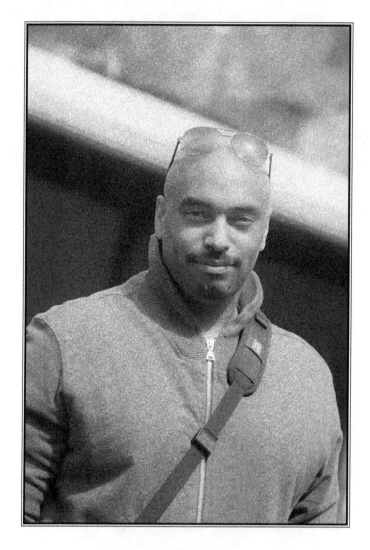

"Dino"
Son

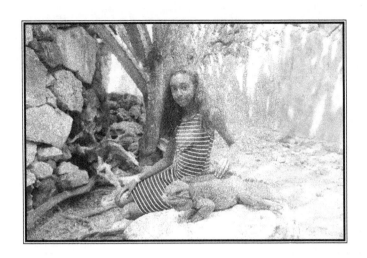

"Cierra Raine"
Grand-daughter

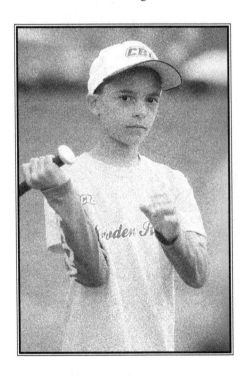

"Chase Alexander"
Grandson

NOTES

NOTES

About the Author

Angella Dixon-Watson is a pancreatic cancer survivor. She is passionate about spreading awareness of pancreatic cancer and its subtlety.

She started experiencing itching in the palm of her hands, which graduated to her entire body, except her face; became jaundiced and had rapid weight loss within a four week period. These symptoms could have meant any other illness but since she did not have expertise in the medical field, she immediately sought medical attention.

Angella is encouraging you to pay attention to your bodies "It speaks to us!" Only about 15 percent diagnosed with pancreatic cancer makes it to surgery. Her hope is that with more funding and research for early detection, the survival rate will be greater than 10%.

Her desire is that you will be encouraged from scriptural and song references throughout her journal and for you to hold on to HOPE.

Angella grew up in a Christian home in Jamaica, where she learned the values of trust and faith; spending early mornings in worship before heading off to Harrison Memorial High School.

She graduated from Northern Caribbean and Washington Adventist Universities. Her main career path was working in administration at both the World Bank and the International Monetary Fund (IMF).

She has two children Roosevelt Dilano and Raquel-Ann. Her two grandchildren are Cierra Raine and Chase Alexander Burke. Her husband is Ira Watson.

CPSIA information can be obtained
at www.ICGtesting.com
Printed in the USA
LVHW02s1045060518
576190LV00002B/144/P